LACTOSE INTOLERANCE DIET PLAN GUIDE BOOK

Lactose Intolerant Diet: Mouthwatering Recipes and Expert Tips

REX LEWIS

Table of Contents

Introduction 4

CHAPTER ONE..........................9

What Is Lactose Intolerance?........9

Clinical Manifestations And Identification 12

Incidence and Determinants 17

CHAPTER TWO.......................21

Role of Lactose In The Body........21

Establishing a Kitchen Free Of Lactose 24

CHAPTER THREE 30

Nutrition and Lactose Intolerance 30

Lactose-Free Meal Planning........36

CHAPTER FOUR.....................42

Addressing Lactose Intolerance across Various Life Phases 42

Conclusion 49

THE END 52

Introduction

Lactose Intolerance Is A Prevalent Digestive Illness Characterized By The Body's Inability To Completely Digest Lactose, A Sugar Present In Milk And Dairy Products. Lactase Insufficiency Causes The Inability To Break Down Lactose Into Glucose And Galactose Due To A Lack Of The Enzyme Lactase Generated In The Small Intestine.

People With Lactose Intolerance May Suffer From Symptoms Like Bloating, Flatulence, Diarrhea, And Abdominal Pain Following The Use Of Dairy Products. Lactose Intolerance, Although Not Life-Threatening, Can

Greatly Affect An Individual's Quality Of Life.

To Manage Lactose Intolerance, One Must Follow A Lactose Intolerance Diet That Aims To Reduce Or Eliminate The Consumption Of Foods Containing Lactose. Here Are Some Overarching Principles For A Lactose Intolerance Diet:

• Choose Lactose-Free Or Low-Lactose Options Such Lactose-Free Milk, Cheese, And Yogurt As Alternatives To Regular Dairy Products. These Items Have Undergone A Process To Hydrolyze Lactose, Rendering Them More Digestible.

- **Non-Dairy Alternatives:** Consider Non-Dairy Options Like Almond Milk, Soy Milk, Coconut Milk, Or Plant-Based Lactose-Free Milk. These Options Are Versatile For Use In Cooking, Baking, And As A Drink.

- Hard And Matured Cheeses, Such As Cheddar Or Swiss, Typically Include Less Lactose Than Fresh Cheeses. These May Be More Easily Digested By Persons With Lactose Sensitivity.

- Consider Taking Lactase Supplements Prior To Consuming Dairy Products. These Supplements Include The Enzyme That Is Lacking In The Body, Aiding In The More Efficient Breakdown Of Lactose.

• Be Vigilant Of Concealed Sources Of Lactose: Lactose May Be Found In A Variety Of Processed Foods, Pharmaceuticals, And Even In Some Surprising Sources. Examine Ingredient Lists For Words Such As Whey, Curds, Milk By-Products, Dry Milk Solids, And Non-Fat Dry Milk Powder.

• **Gradual Introduction:** Some People With Lactose Intolerance Can Handle Tiny Quantities Of Lactose Without Experiencing Symptoms. Slowly Incorporate Dairy Back Into Your Diet In Modest Amounts And Monitor How Your Body Reacts.

Individuals With Lactose Intolerance Should Customize Their Diet

According To Their Personal Tolerances And Preferences. Seeking Advice From A Healthcare Expert Or A Trained Dietitian Can Offer Specific Recommendations To Maintain Proper Nutrition While Dealing With Lactose Intolerance.

CHAPTER ONE
What Is Lactose Intolerance?

Lactose Intolerance Is A Digestive Condition When The Body Is Unable To Completely Digest Lactose, A Sugar Present In Milk And Dairy Products. Lactase Insufficiency Causes The Inability To Break Down Lactose Into Glucose And Galactose Due To A Lack Of The Enzyme Lactase Generated In The Small Intestine.

• If There Is Not Enough Lactase, Lactose Cannot Be Properly Digested In The Intestine, Causing Discomfort When Consuming Meals That Contain Lactose. The Symptoms Usually Consist Of Bloating, Flatulence, Stomach Pain, Diarrhea, And

Occasionally Nausea. Symptom Severity Can Vary Significantly Among Individuals And May Be Influenced By Factors Including The Quantity Of Lactose Ingested And The Extent Of Lactase Insufficiency.

• Lactose Intolerance Can Manifest At Any Age But Is Typically Observed Throughout Adolescence Or Maturity. It Can Result From Genetic Factors Leading To Decreased Lactase Production With Age Or From Damage To The Small Intestine Caused By Infections, Gastrointestinal Illnesses, Or Specific Medicinal Treatments.

• Lactose Intolerance Should Be Distinguished From A Milk Allergy. Lactose Intolerance Is Characterized

By Challenges In Digesting Lactose, Whereas A Milk Allergy Is An Immune System Reaction To The Proteins Present In Milk And Dairy Items, Resulting In Allergic Responses That Vary In Severity.

Lactose Intolerance, While Not Life-Threatening, Can Greatly Affect A Person's Quality Of Life. To Manage Lactose Intolerance, Individuals Usually Make Dietary Changes By Minimizing Or Eliminating Lactose-Containing Meals, Opting For Lactose-Free Options, And Occasionally Using Lactase Supplements To Assist With Digestion. Seeking Advice From A Healthcare Expert Or A Certified Dietician Might Offer Tailored

Assistance In Properly Managing Lactose Intolerance.

Clinical Manifestations And Identification

Lactose Intolerance Symptoms Usually Manifest After Ingesting Meals Or Beverages Containing Lactose. Symptom Severity Varies Across Individuals, And Some May Tolerate Tiny Doses Of Lactose Without Pain. Typical Symptoms Consist Of:

• Bloating Occurs When There Is An Accumulation Of Excess Gas In The Digestive Tract, Leading To A Sensation Of Fullness And Bloating.

• Gas Can Be Produced In The Intestines Due To Incomplete

Digestion Of Lactose By The Enzyme Lactase In The Body.

• Abdomen Pain Characterized By Cramping Or Discomfort In The Abdomen Region Is A Prevalent Sign Of Lactose Intolerance.

• Diarrhea May Occur When Undigested Lactose Attracts Water Into The Intestines, Resulting In Loose Stools.

• Nausea May Occur In Some People After Consuming Meals That Contain Lactose.

Differentiating Between Lactose Intolerance And Other Gastrointestinal Diseases With Similar Symptoms Is Crucial. If You Suspect Lactose

Intolerance, A Healthcare Expert May Suggest The Following Diagnostic Methods:

1. Your Doctor Will Ask About Your Symptoms, How Often They Occur, And When They Started In Relation To Ingesting Dairy Products.

2. An Elimination Diet Is A Frequent Approach That Entails Removing Lactose-Containing Foods From Your Diet For A Specific Duration To Determine If Symptoms Alleviate. If Symptoms Improve During The Elimination Phase But Reappear When Lactose Is Reintroduced, It Could Indicate Lactose Intolerance.

3. The Hydrogen Breath Test Is A Non-Invasive Procedure That Quantifies The Hydrogen Levels In Your Breath Following The Ingestion Of A Lactose-Based Solution. Bacteria Ferment Undigested Lactose In The Colon, Creating Hydrogen, Which Is Taken Into The Circulation And Expelled.

4. Stool Acidity Test: This Test Assesses The Acidity Of The Stool Following Lactose Consumption. Unprocessed Lactose In The Colon Might Elevate The Acidity Of The Feces.

5. A Lactose Tolerance Test Requires Consuming A Beverage With Lactose And Monitoring Blood Glucose Levels Periodically. Normal Individuals See

An Increase In Blood Glucose Levels Following Lactose Eating Due To Adequate Lactase Levels. Yet, In Individuals With Lactose Sensitivity, The Increase Is Small.

It Is Essential To Get Advice From A Healthcare Professional For A Precise Diagnosis And Suitable Treatment. Once Lactose Intolerance Is Diagnosed, Dietary Modifications, Lactase Supplements, And Other Techniques Can Be Suggested To Effectively Control Symptoms.

Incidence and Determinants

Lactose Intolerance Is A Widespread Disorder Globally, With Varying Prevalence Rates Across Different Communities And Ethnicities. Factors Affecting The Prevalence Of Lactose Intolerance Include:

• Some Ethnic Groups Have A Higher Prevalence Of Lactose Intolerance Due To Genetics. It Is Prevalent Among Individuals Of African, Asian, Native American, And Hispanic Origin. Individuals Of Northern European Ancestry Typically Exhibit A Reduced Occurrence Of Lactose Intolerance. Genetic Factors Greatly Influence An Individual's Capacity To Make Lactase Into Maturity.

• Lactose Intolerance Can Manifest At Any Age, However It Is Typically More Prevalent In Adolescence And Maturity. Infants And Early Children Often Have Enough Lactase To Break Down Breast Milk Or Formula, But Some People May Generate Less Lactase As They Get Older.

• Geography Plays A Role In The Varying Rates Of Lactose Intolerance. Regions Like Northern Europe, Where Dairy Consumption Has Been Traditionally High, Tend To Have Lower Rates Of Lactose Intolerance Compared To Regions With Lower Historical Dairy Consumption.

• Medical Diseases And Gastrointestinal Issues Can Cause

Secondary Lactose Intolerance. Various Disorders That Impact The Small Intestine, Such As Infections, Celiac Disease, And Crohn's Disease, Can Lead To A Decrease In Lactase Production.

• Medications And Therapies Like Chemotherapy Can Impact Lactase Production And Lead To Lactose Intolerance.

• Premature Newborns May Experience Transient Lactose Intolerance Due To Reduced Amounts Of Lactase. Lactase Production Often Rises As The Infant Develops.

Lactose Intolerance Is Not A Binary Condition. People Can Have Different

Levels Of Lactose Intolerance, And Others May Tolerate Modest Quantities Of Lactose Without Experiencing Symptoms. The Occurrence Of Lactose Intolerance May Vary Throughout Time Due To Influences Like Dietary Choices And Lifestyle Habits.

Individuals Who Suspect Lactose Intolerance Or Have Symptoms After Consuming Dairy Products Should Get Advice From A Healthcare Expert. A Healthcare Provider Can Perform Diagnostic Tests And Offer Advice On Efficiently Treating Lactose Intolerance.

CHAPTER TWO
Role of Lactose In The Body

Lactose Functions As An Energy And Nutritional Source, Especially In Infancy, Where It Plays A Vital Role In Mammalian Milk, Such As Human Breast Milk. Lactose's Main Role In The Body Is To Serve As A Readily Accessible Energy Source For Developing Organisms, Particularly Babies. Here Are Some Primary Roles Of Lactose:

• **Energy Source:** Lactose Is A Disaccharide Sugar Made Up Of Glucose And Galactose. Lactose Is Transformed Into Simpler Sugars By The Enzyme Lactase In The Small Intestine, Allowing For Absorption

Into The Bloodstream. Glucose Is The Main Energy Source For Cells, And Galactose Can Be Transformed Into Glucose To Provide Energy.

• Lactose Is Required For The Absorption Of Important Nutrients, Such As Calcium. Calcium Is Essential For The Growth And Upkeep Of Healthy Bones And Teeth. Without Lactose Or In Cases Of Lactose Sensitivity, Individuals May Struggle To Get Enough Calcium From Dairy Products, Which Could Affect Bone Health.

• Lactose Acts As A Substrate For The Growth Of Beneficial Bacteria In The Colon, Like Bifidobacteria. The Bacteria Help Maintain A Healthy

Balance Of Microflora In The Gastrointestinal System, Which Is Essential For General Digestive Health.

• Lactose Is Helpful For Newborns And Young Mammals, But Some Individuals Can Acquire Lactose Intolerance As They Get Older. In Certain Instances, The Body Does Not Create Enough Of The Enzyme Lactase Required To Metabolize Lactose, Resulting In Challenges Digesting Dairy Products.

Individuals With Lactose Intolerance Can Effectively Manage Their Diet By Opting For Lactose-Free Or Low-Lactose Alternatives, Taking Lactase Supplements, And Ensuring They Get Essential Nutrients From Other Food Sources Despite Challenges In

Obtaining Nutrients From Dairy Products. Lactose Intolerance Generally Does Not Present A Substantial Health Threat, And Individuals With This Condition Can Maintain A Healthy Lifestyle By Making Suitable Dietary Modifications.

Establishing a Kitchen Free Of Lactose

To Establish A Lactose-Free Kitchen, One Must Carefully Select Ingredients, Cooking Techniques, And Food Preparation Procedures To Cater To Persons With Lactose Sensitivity. Here Are Some Guidelines To Assist You In Setting Up A Lactose-Free Kitchen:

1. Opt For Lactose-Free Options.

• Choose Lactose-Free Dairy Products Such As Milk, Cheese, And Yogurt. Several Supermarket Stores Provide Lactose-Free Alternatives For These Products.

• Investigate Non-Dairy Options Including Almond Milk, Soy Milk, Coconut Milk, And Oat Milk As Substitutes For Conventional Dairy Products.

2. Review The Labels:

• Examine Ingredient Labels Thoroughly To Detect Lactose-Containing Components In Packaged And Processed Foods. Beware Of Ingredients Such As Whey, Curds, Milk

By-Products, Dry Milk Solids, And Non-Fat Dry Milk Powder.

3. Stock Your Pantry With Lactose-Free Essentials.

• Ensure Your Cupboard Is Supplied With Lactose-Free Replacements For Typical Dairy Ingredients, Like Lactose-Free Milk, Butter, And Cheese Substitutes.

4. Utilize Non-Dairy Cooking Fats.

• Substitute Traditional Butter With Lactose-Free Margarine Or Non-Dairy Alternatives Such As Olive Oil, Coconut Oil, Or Vegetable Oil In Your Cooking And Baking.

5. Explore Lactose-Free Recipes:

• Discover Recipes Tailored For Persons With Lactose Intolerance. Various Websites And Cookbooks Provide Innovative And Tasty Lactose-Free Recipes.

6. Be Aware Of Concealed Lactose.

• Be Cautious Of Concealed Sources Of Lactose In Surprising Locations, Like Pharmaceuticals, Salad Dressings, And Processed Meals. Verify Labels Or Seek Advice From A Pharmacist To Confirm Drugs Are Free Of Lactose.

7. Use Fresh And Unprocessed Foods.

• Prioritize Incorporating Fresh, Healthful Foods Into Your Meals.

Fruits, Vegetables, Lean Proteins, Grains, And Legumes Are Inherently Lactose-Free And Can Serve As The Foundation Of A Nutritious Diet.

8. Consider Investing In Lactase Supplements.

• Consider Keeping Lactase Supplements Available. These Supplements Can Be Given Prior To Eating Foods That Might Have Concealed Lactose, Enabling Those With Lactose Sensitivity To Consume Some Dairy Products More Comfortably.

9. Teach Family Members:

• Inform Family Members Or Housemates About Lactose

Intolerance And The Necessity Of Having Lactose-Free Options In The Kitchen If You Share It With Others.

10. Establish A Distinct Storage Area: Consider Creating A Dedicated Space In The Kitchen For Lactose-Free Items To Prevent Cross-Contamination With Products Containing Lactose.

By Implementing These Ideas, You Can Establish A Lactose-Free Kitchen That Caters To The Nutritional Requirements Of Those With Lactose Intolerance While Still Offering A Varied And Pleasurable Selection Of Meals And Snacks.

CHAPTER THREE
Nutrition and Lactose Intolerance

To Manage Lactose Intolerance Effectively, Individuals Need To Focus On Nutrition To Get Vital Nutrients While Reducing Symptoms Caused By Consuming Lactose. Here Are Important Factors To Consider For Keeping Proper Nutrition When Dealing With Lactose Intolerance:

1. Select Lactose-Free Options.

• Choose Lactose-Free Alternatives For Milk, Cheese, Yogurt, And Other Dairy Items. These Alternatives Have Been Processed To Hydrolyze Lactose, Facilitating Digestion.

2. Investigate Non-Dairy Options.

• Incorporate Non-Dairy Options Like Almond Milk, Soy Milk, Coconut Milk, And Oat Milk Into Your Diet. These Substitutes Are Frequently Enriched With Vitamins And Minerals Like Calcium And Vitamin D To Replicate The Nutritional Content Of Dairy Products.

3. Choose From Lactose-Free Or Hard Cheeses.

• Hard And Matured Cheeses Like Cheddar Or Swiss Typically Have Reduced Lactose Levels And May Be More Easily Digested By People With Lactose Intolerance.

4. Ensure Sufficient Calcium Consumption.

• Since Dairy Is A Major Calcium Source, It Is Crucial To Acquire This Critical Mineral From Alternative Sources. Incorporate Calcium-Rich Foods Into Your Diet, Such As Leafy Green Vegetables (Kale, Broccoli), Fortified Non-Dairy Milks, Tofu, And Tinned Fish With Bones (Such As Salmon Or Sardines).

5. List Vitamin D Sources:

• Vitamin D Is Crucial For The Absorption Of Calcium. Incorporate Vitamin D Sources Into Your Diet, Such As Fatty Fish (Salmon, Mackerel), Egg Yolks, And Vitamin D-Fortified Foods

Like Certain Cereals And Non-Dairy Milks.

6. Eat Foods That Are Rich In Probiotics.

• Probiotics Are Advantageous For Intestinal Health. Incorporate Probiotic-Rich Foods Like Yogurt Substitutes Containing Live Cultures, Kefir, Sauerkraut, And Kimchi Into Your Diet.

7. Track Dietary Fiber Consumption.

• Some People With Lactose Intolerance May Have Alterations In Their Bowel Movements. Consume Sufficient Fiber From Fruits,

Vegetables, Whole Grains, And Legumes To Support Digestive Health.

8. Enhance With Lactase Enzymes:

• Consider Using Lactase Supplements Before To Consuming Dairy Products To Aid In The Breakdown Of Lactose. This Is Particularly Beneficial When Desiring To Consume Small Quantities Of Lactose-Containing Meals.

9. Keep Yourself Well-Hydrated.

• Lactose Intolerance Symptoms May Result In Dehydration, Particularly If Diarrhea Is A Frequent Symptom. Stay Hydrated By Consuming Ample Amounts Of Water.

10. Seek Advice From A Nutrition Specialist.

• Consult A Certified Dietitian Or Healthcare Professional To Develop A Customized Nutrition Plan Tailored To Your Specific Requirements, Guaranteeing A Well-Rounded And Nutrient-Dense Diet.

Maintaining A Diverse And Balanced Diet Is Crucial For Meeting Nutritional Requirements When Dealing With Lactose Intolerance. Seeking Guidance From A Healthcare Expert Or Dietician Can Offer Personalized Recommendations Considering Individual Tastes, Tolerances, And Nutritional Needs.

Lactose-Free Meal Planning

Planning Meals For Those With Lactose Sensitivity Requires Selecting Lactose-Free Or Low-Lactose Items To Maintain A Balanced And Nutritious Diet. Here Is A Lactose-Free Meal Planning Guide.

First Meal of the Day:

1. Make Oats Using Lactose-Free Milk Or A Non-Dairy Substitute.

• Top The Dish With Fresh Berries, Sliced Bananas, Or Other Fruits.

• Sprinkle Nuts Or Seeds For Extra Crunch.

2. Prepare A Smoothie Bowl By Blending Lactose-Free Yogurt

Substitute With Frozen Berries, Banana, And A Dash Of Lactose-Free Milk.

• Top The Dish With Granola, Shredded Coconut, And Chia Seeds.

3. Prepare An Egg And Vegetable Scramble By Mixing Eggs With Spinach, Tomatoes, And Bell Peppers.

• Pair With Whole-Grain Bread And Avocado.

Lunch:

1. Grilled Chicken Salad: Grilled Chicken Mixed With Assorted Greens, Cherry Tomatoes, Cucumber, And Olives.

• Coat With Olive Oil And Balsamic Vinegar.

2. Prepare A Quinoa And Vegetable Bowl By Cooking Quinoa And Mixing It With Roasted Zucchini, Bell Peppers, And Cherry Tomatoes.

• Drizzle With Lemon Vinaigrette And Add Grilled Tofu Or Chicken On Top.

3. Make A Robust Lentil Soup With Carrots, Celery, And Spices.

• Serve With Gluten-Free Crackers On The Side.

Dinner:

1. Baked Salmon With Lemon Herb Sauce: - Bake Salmon And Top With A

Sauce Consisting Of Lemon Juice, Olive Oil, And Fresh Herbs.

• Pair With Steamed Asparagus And Quinoa.

2. Prepare A Vegetarian Stir-Fry By Cooking Tofu With Broccoli, Snap Peas, Carrots, And Bell Peppers.

• Serve Over Rice Or Rice Noodles With A Soy Sauce Alternative.

• Create A Robust Chili Using Ground Turkey, Sweet Potatoes, Tomatoes, And Kidney Beans.

• Top With Vegan Cheese Or Avocado.

Snacks:

1. Enjoy Sliced Apples Or Bananas With Almond Butter Or Peanut Butter For A Fresh Fruit Snack.

2. Opt For A Lactose-Free Or Plant-Based Yogurt In Greek Style. Serve With Granola And Assorted Fruit.

3. Prepare Air-Popped Popcorn And Season With Nutritional Yeast For A Tasty Snack.

Desserts:

1. Fruit Sorbet: Enjoy A Revitalizing Sorbet Crafted From Blended Frozen Fruit.

• Decorate With Mint Leaves.

2. Prepare A Dairy-Free Chocolate Mousse By Blending Ripe Avocados With Cocoa Powder And Sugar.

3. Make Coconut Milk Rice Pudding By Cooking Rice In Coconut Milk And Sweetening It With Sugar Or A Sugar Substitute.

• Sprinkle Cinnamon on Top.

Be Sure To Carefully Read Labels To Find Hidden Sources Of Lactose In Packaged Foods, And Adjust These Meal Suggestions According To Your Tastes And Dietary Needs. When Uncertain, Seeking Advice From A Trained Dietitian Can Offer Tailored Direction For A Lactose-Free Eating Plan.

CHAPTER FOUR
Addressing Lactose Intolerance across Various Life Phases

Managing Lactose Intolerance Might Differ Depending On The Life Cycle, And Modifications May Be Required To Accommodate The Evolving Dietary Requirements Of Individuals. Here Are Factors To Consider When Managing Lactose Intolerance At Various Life Stages:

1. Early Stages of Development:

• Infants Can Usually Metabolize Lactose Present In Breast Milk Or Formula. If You Suspect Lactose Intolerance, Seek Help From A Pediatrician.

• During Childhood, Progressively Introduce Foods Containing Lactose To Observe Tolerance. It Is Important To Regularly Assess For The Development Of Lactose Intolerance Later In Life.

2. Adolescence:

• Lactose Intolerance May Develop In Adolescents During This Stage. Symptoms May Intensify, Necessitating Dietary Modifications.

• Make Sure To Get Enough Calcium From Other Sources If You Don't Consume Dairy Products. Fortified Plant-Based Milks, Leafy Greens, And Tofu Are Advantageous Non-Dairy Sources.

3. Young Adulthood:

• Lactose Intolerance Is Frequently Identified Throughout The Young Adult Years. Explore Lactose-Free Options To Find Appropriate Replacements For Preferred Dairy Items.

• When Ingesting Modest Amounts Of Lactose-Containing Foods, It Is Advisable To Consider Using Lactase Supplements.

4. Pregnancy Can Impact Lactose Tolerance. Temporary Lactose Intolerance In Some Women During Pregnancy Can Be Attributed To Hormonal Fluctuations.

• Consume Sufficient Calcium From Non-Dairy Sources, Particularly If Experiencing Lactose Intolerance Symptoms When Pregnant Or Breastfeeding.

5. Adulthood:

• Lactose Intolerance Is Frequently Identified In Adulthood. Select Lactose-Free Or Low-Lactose Options And Keep Track Of Your Tolerance Levels.

• Prioritize A Balanced Diet High In Nutrients From Non-Dairy Sources To Sustain General Well-Being.

6. As Individuals Age, They Often See A Decline In Lactase Synthesis, Resulting

In A Higher Occurrence Of Lactose Intolerance Among Older Persons.

• Emphasize Consuming Foods High In Calcium And Contemplate Using Supplements If Necessary, As Preserving Bone Health Becomes Essential.

7. Postmenopause:

• Menopausal Hormonal Changes Can Affect Lactose Tolerance. Some Women May Have Reduced Lactase Production.

• Monitor Symptoms, Alter Diet As Needed, And Maintain Sufficient Nutritional Intake For Overall Health.

8. Senior Years:

• Aging Can Lead To A Reduction In Lactase Production. Monitor Symptoms And Modify Diet To Control Lactose Intolerance. Prioritize Nutrient-Rich Foods To Fulfill Dietary Needs, Particularly Calcium And Vitamin D For Bone Health.

At Various Life Phases, It Is Important To Be Aware Of Personal Tolerance Levels, Adapt Food Selections Accordingly, And Consult Healthcare Professionals Or Dietitians For Tailored Recommendations. Consistent Evaluations, A Well-Rounded Diet, And Suitable Supplementation When Necessary Can Assist Individuals In Efficiently

Handling Lactose Intolerance At All Stages Of Life.

Conclusion

Ultimately, Handling Lactose Intolerance Requires A Mix Of Dietary Modifications, Selective Food Selections, And Potentially Supplement Usage. Lactose Intolerance Is A Prevalent Digestive Ailment That Can Impact People At Different Points In Their Lives. It Is Essential To Comprehend And Manage Lactose Intolerance From Early Childhood To Old Age To Uphold Good Health And Wellness.

Following A Lactose-Free Diet Necessitates Individuals To Carefully Select Their Food Options, Choosing Lactose-Free Substitutes And Making Well-Informed Selections While Eating

Out. It Is Crucial To Inform Restaurant Personnel About Dietary Requirements And To Be Mindful Of Concealed Lactose Sources In Packaged And Processed Foods.

Ensuring A Diet That Is Both Balanced And Rich In Nutrients Is Crucial For Achieving Nutritional Needs, Particularly In Cases When Dairy Consumption Is Restricted. Highlighting Other Sources Of Calcium, Vitamin D, And Other Vital Nutrients Is Crucial For Those With Lactose Intolerance To Sustain Good Health.

With Advancements In Technology And Food Choices, Those Who Are Lactose Intolerant Now Have A Wider Range Of Lactose-Free Products And

Alternative Nutrient Sources Available To Them. Seeking Advice From Healthcare Professionals Or Trained Dietitians Can Offer Tailored Assistance And Encouragement For Properly Handling Lactose Intolerance At Various Life Stages.

Individuals With Lactose Intolerance Can Live Full And Productive Lives By Making Informed Dietary Choices, Advocating For Their Needs, And Embracing A Variety Of Lactose-Free And Nutritious Foods.

THE END